WOMEN AND THE MIDLIFE EXPERIENCE:
WHEN THE GLASS SLIPPER NO LONGER FITS

A Workbook for Busy Women

Second edition

DONNA SELL KOHLHEPP, PH.D., RN
And
JAYNE M. MAGEE, PH.D.

TABLE OF CONTENTS

Preface

Since we originally wrote this workbook, there have been many new developments in the health care field concerning women, midlife, and menopause. More research on women's health issues is being done daily. This is encouraging. Prior to this era, most all the major medical research was being done on men.

We are two Baby Boomers. When we started writing this workbook, both of us were in perimenopause. Now, both of us have passed on to postmenopause, and one of us is a breast cancer survivor. Our daughters are headed into midlife, and their lives are very different from ours. Menopause is no longer a "dirty word" or "the curse." Our daughters report that women their age talk about everything, so it was time to bring this workbook into the 21st century.

We have new information and insights to share. However, what has surprised us the most is just how timely and relevant much of what we published in the first edition still is. So we kept what was good, solid content, but we have updated it with new resources (see Section 4), new research and treatments, and our own accumulated wisdom. We also added a section on male menopause for women to understand and appreciation that their men, too, are going through changes at this age.

Pour yourself a glass of wine or a cup of coffee, open up a box of chocolate, find a quiet and peaceful spot, and give yourself permission to relax, refresh, and renew as you read this workbook. The beauty of this format is that you don't need to read it front to back like a textbook. You can flip it open to any page and learn something new or find confirmation that you are, indeed, in the best place in your life right now.

Introduction

Women and the Midlife Experience: When the Glass Slipper No Longer Fits is an informative and supportive workbook for women anticipating the midlife passage, as well as for women who are searching for an understanding of the changes and choices in midlife that they are experiencing. It offers a holistic approach to women's health and wellness issues. The title of this book is a metaphor for the midlife experience of giving up our fairytale image of women as helpless Cinderellas and recognizing the myths and stereotypes concerning women. This book is an attempt to expose the myths surrounding the aging process and contrast them with the facts. Midlife is a time for discarding the glass slipper that no longer fits because of our swollen feet and changing lifestyles. It is a time for assembling the pieces of our lives--the roles we played, the people we used to be, the people we are becoming, the physical, emotional, and psychological changes we experience at midlife to create a beautiful "patchwork quilt."

In **Section One**, we discuss physical changes that in occur in midlife as a result of menopause. What are the realities, and what are the myths associated with midlife, menopausal women? What is menopause and what is it not? Conditions that might be confused with menopause are ruled out.   Common complaints and concerns associated with menopause are identified, as well as suggestions for how women can manage them.   The risks and benefits of hormone replacement therapy are presented, as well as additional remedies and alternative approaches such a supplements and lifestyle changes. This section also discusses important midlife health issues other than menopause: heart disease, osteoporosis, and breast cancer.

In **Section Two**, the focus is on the emotional and psychological concerns of midlife, including life changes and losses, and blue funk or malaise. We also examine midlife as a Grief Process, including moving forward to the reinvestment of our time and energy to prepare for the opportunities our futures hold.

The workbook format provides for and encourages group discussion for better understanding the midlife experience. Each section includes

Journal Prompts/ Discussion Questions for those who wish to further explore the issues raised in the chapters. Many women find journaling or writing a useful tool in dealing with concerns and feelings while others may find talking with others valuable. The Journal Prompts/ Discussion Questions are meant to help you focus on the issues.

By presenting facts and suggestions for coping with the changes and choices of midlife, we hope to dismiss the myths characterizing midlife as a negative state to be dreaded and treated. Instead, midlife can be seen as a time of change and opportunity.

SECTION ONE:
Physical Changes in Midlife

WHAT MENOPAUSE IS AND WHAT IT IS NOT

The word menopause is generally used in reference to the phase of the aging process of women marking the transition from the reproductive state of life to the non-reproductive state. More specifically, menopause refers to the single point in time of the last menstrual period. The phase before the last period is referred to as perimenopause, and the phase after is referred to as postmenopause. Each phase is associated with different characteristics and different hormone levels.

Menopause is often seen as a time of life to be dreaded. It has been referred to as "the curse," and it is surrounded by negative myths
The actual facts of menopause give a much more accurate and more positive view of this stage of life. Some of these facts may surprise you.

Myths of Menopause:

- *Menopause marks the beginning of a downhill slide.*

- *Post menopause is an estrogen-deficient state in need of treatment.*

- *Menopausal women are sexless undesirable, melancholic, neurotic, insane, hypochondriacs.*

Facts of Menopause:

- *The average age of menopause is 51 years.*

- *Women who start menstruation early tend to finish late; and those who start menstruation late, tend to finish early. This seems to be the opposite of what might be expected.*

- *Left-handed women tend to have an earlier menopause.*

- *Smoking, stresses, and other illnesses can lead to an earlier menopause.*

- *Late-in- life pregnancies can lead to an early menopause. In fact, some women after having a baby in their late thirties or forties may never resume having periods after delivery.*

- *Women who suffer from PMS tend to have a later menopause.*

- *There is a familial similarity in the timing of menopause. In other words, our age of menopause is similar to that of our mother's and sisters.'*

- *Seventy-five to eighty percent of women will develop symptoms due to hormone fluctuations during perimenopause. However, some women may never become symptomatic because they produce hormones over a longer period of time and have a slower waning of the process.*

- *Women with more fat store more estrogen during menopause, and therefore tend to have fewer symptoms. Some have suggested that this is the reason women tend to put on weight during perimenopause. It may be the body's way of taking care of its needs for estrogen during this period of decreasing hormone production. So enjoy those extra pounds!*

- *Estrogen levels do not fall to zero after menopause; they merely remain lower than necessary for the monthly cycle. However, progesterone levels do fall to nearly zero.*

- *More and more contemporary literature and media reports suggest that American women who have reached menopause say they are happier and more fulfilled than when they were younger   As our friend and mother-in-law Jackie Kohlhepp once said, " Midlife is the cocktail hour of our lives."*

Aging vs. menopause

Menopause is not the same as normal aging. We all age, men and women alike. Not all changes are a result of hormones. Below is a list of the common signs of aging.

- Skin changes such as thinning and wrinkles
- Joint stiffness
- Loss of flexibility
- Increased recovery time after activity
- Loss of hair pigment (graying)
- Loss of flexibility of visual focus (far sightedness)
- Slower reaction time and memory
- Weight gain

<u>We cannot blame everything on menopause or expect to prevent aging by trying to treat it or prevent it.</u>

Facts:
- *Although there are changes and losses as we age, it need not be seen as a straight downhill slide.*

- *Aging is not a loss of intelligence or the beginning of senility. In fact, only 4% of men or women develop true senility.*

- *We become better conceptual learners as we age, as well as more socially intelligent.*

- *The eyes' ability to accommodate for distance starts diminishing at the age of 10, but it is not noticeable until about age 40. The loss of flexibility of visual focus is usually fixed by age 55 or 60.   In other words, we won't necessarily need to continue getting stronger and stronger glasses as we age.*

- *Many of the changes related to aging can be slowed or improved with a healthy lifestyle.*

The facts are encouraging. We can look forward to being smarter in some respects and more socially capable. It is also encouraging to know that we do have some control over how we age with our lifestyle choices.

JOURNAL PROMPTS/ DISCUSSION QUESTIONS:
WHAT MENOPAUSE IS AND WHAT IT IS NOT

- ✓ List words you associate with the following:
    - <u>young woman</u>
    - <u>young man</u>
    - <u>middle-aged woman</u>
    - <u>middle-aged man</u>
    - <u>menopause</u>
    - <u>old woman</u>
    - <u>old man</u>

- ✓ Reread your list of words above. How have these images shaped your own expectations of the midlife experience?

- ✓ Where have these images come from? (Hint: media, magazines, movies, social media, fairy tales, etc)?

- ✓ Are these realistic images?

- ✓ Would you have listed the same words that you wrote in the first prompt tens years ago? If not why?

HORMONAL PHASES

Perimenopause

Perimenopause describes the years of gradual hormonal change before the last menstrual period. It can begin as early as 35 years, or it can be delayed as late as 50 years and last as long as 10 years. On average, the phase occurs somewhere between ages 45 and 55, and lasts 4 years.

The female hormones that are responsible for the monthly cycle include estrogen, progesterone, lutenizing hormone (LH), and follicle-stimulating hormone (FSH). After puberty, these hormones work in harmony increasing and decreasing at the appropriate times of the month. This allows for the preparation of the uterine lining and the release of an egg for possible fertilization or eventual menstruation.

As we age, there is a decrease in the number of viable eggs released from the ovary. Some months an egg will be released, and other months one will not until eventually there are no more eggs. This marks the end of fertility. Along with the decrease in fertility, there is also a change in the hormone levels. The changes are similar to those in puberty, only in reverse. Ideally, in perimenopause estrogen levels gradually decline along with progesterone levels with some increase in the lutenizing and follicle-stimulating hormone. For some, this change occurs without symptoms. More commonly, for about 80% of women, the hormones get out of balance for a time resulting in discomforts.

A list of common signs and symptoms associated with the hormonal changes of menopause follows.

Common signs and symptoms of hormonal change:
- _____ Hot flashes, flushes, night sweats
- _____ Bouts of rapid heart beat, heart palpitations
- _____ Irritability
- _____ Mood swings, sudden tears
- _____ Trouble sleeping through the night (with or without sweats)
- _____ Crashing fatigue
- _____ Loss of libido (sexual desire)
- _____ Anxiety, feeling ill at ease, paranoia
- _____ Feelings of dread, apprehension, doom

_____ Irregular periods: shorter, lighter periods; heavier periods; flooding
_____ Weight gain 10-15 pounds
_____ Sudden bouts of bloating
_____ Vaginal dryness
_____ Itchy, creepy, crawly skin sensations
_____ Aching, sore joints and muscles
_____ Breast changes: tenderness and/or sagging
_____ Headache change: increase or decrease
_____ Difficulty concentrating, disorientation, confusion
_____ Disturbing memory lapses
_____ Depression
_____ Bladder changes, incontinence: especially upon sneezing or laughing
_____ Gum problems, bleeding gums
_____ Heat intolerance
_____ Carpal Tunnel Syndrome
_____ Numbness of hands and feet
_____ Recurrent vaginal infections
_____ Recurrent bladder infections

This list of complaints is extensive and there can be others. Often existing conditions get worse. Women report changes in digestion, such as heartburn or gas. Others report changes in their allergies: some get better others have increased symptoms and problems with asthma. There is also something some postmenopausal women suffer with called "idiopathic-post-nasal drip." Idiopathic means they do not have an explanation as to why it occurs. As hormone levels change with menopause, there is a change in the body's chemistry that has an effect throughout the entire body, not just the reproductive system.   But remember, no one has all of the symptoms, and most will resolve when the hormones rebalance after menopause. Sometimes it is just reassuring to see that what you are experiencing is not abnormal, life threatening, or uncommon.

<u>Alternative Explanations for Symptoms</u>
Many of the symptoms of hormone change are similar to those of other disorders. Hormone changes may merely exacerbate existing conditions and may not necessarily be the cause. It is important to correctly identify the cause of symptoms so that treatment is appropriate. Two conditions that are

often associated with hormone changes include low thyroid and candida
(yeast infections, vaginally or systemically.)

Hypothyroidism: Low thyroid

The thyroid gland is a small gland in the base of the throat that
regulates metabolism. Some estimate that as high as 40% of the
population has undiagnosed, thyroid problems. Thyroid problems
often occur following periods of stress and change and commonly
occur during periods of hormone change. It has been suggested that
postpartum depression may actually be a result of low thyroid levels.
Thyroid issues should be ruled out before assuming that changes or
discomforts are strictly menopausal. As you can see from the list on
the following page, many of the symptoms of low thyroid are similar
to those associated with menopause.

Checklist for Low Thyroid
(*Check the symptoms that you experience. Five or more may be an
indication of low thyroid.*)
_____ Fatigue, low energy level
_____ Difficulty getting up in the morning
_____ Muscle weakness
_____ Feeling cold from the inside out
_____ Abnormally slow pulse
_____ Low blood pressure
_____ Forgetfulness
_____ Difficulty concentrating, slow mental activity
_____ Nervousness
_____ Cold hands and feet
_____ Loss of appetite, difficulty losing weight
_____ Fluid retention
_____ Poor color, or pallor
_____ Dry, scaly skin
_____ Coarse, brittle hair
_____ Thin, brittle nails
_____ Hair loss, dry lifeless hair
_____ Sensitivity to bright light
_____ Yellow bumps on the eyelids
_____ Yellow-orange coloration of the skin (particularly on the palms
        of the hands)

_____ Hoarse voice
_____ Constipation
_____ Depression
_____ Recurrent infections
_____ Elevated cholesterol levels
_____ Decreased libido (sexual desire)
_____ Menstrual difficulties
_____ Early or late puberty (ages 9 or 17)
_____ Fibrocystic disease (breasts cysts or uterine fibroids)
_____ Ovarian cysts
_____ Family history of thyroid disease
_____ Feeling that you just can't cope
_____ Feeling that you just can't keep up like you used to
_____ Morning temperature below 98.2 degrees Fahrenheit

If you have several of the symptoms on the checklist you may want to have your thyroid levels checked by a physician. Most thyroid problems can be diagnosed with a simple blood test. For more information on thyroid disorders see the reference list at the end of the workbook including: Barnes _Hypothyroidism: The Unsuspected Illness_, Wentz _Hashimoto's Thyroiditis_, Hahn _PMS & Menopause: Solving the Puzzle._

Candida Overgrowth

Another condition that can mimic menopause symptoms is Candida overload. Candida overload, Candidiasis, is not always recognized or treated in traditional medicine; however, it is commonly treated by alternative practitioners.

Candida is a yeast that is normally present in our bodies in small amounts. It only becomes a problem when there is an overgrowth. An overgrowth is often a result of the use of antibiotics, hormone therapies, or an abundance of sugar in the diet. Most women are familiar with Candida infections in the mouth, known a thrush, or in the vagina, vaginitis; however, the yeast can settle most anywhere in the body resulting in a wide range of symptoms.

Answer "YES" or "NO" to the following questions.

_____ Do you have diabetes?
_____ Do you have hypoglycemia (low blood sugar)?
_____ Have you had surgery recently?
_____ Have you had recurrent infections?
_____ Do you frequently take antibiotics?
_____ Do you take hormones?
_____ Do have recurrent vaginal infections?
_____ Do eat a lot of sweets?
_____ Do you crave sugar, bread, milk products, or alcohol?
_____ Do you experience gas?
_____ Do you have a white coating on your tongue?
_____ Do you have food allergies?
_____ Do you have bad breath?
_____ Do you have anal itching?
_____ Do you have postnasal drip?
_____ Do you have itchy, scaly skin
_____ Do you experience fluid retention?
_____ Do you have poor coordination?
_____ Do you have difficulty concentrating?
_____ Do you experience foggy thinking, or spaciness?
_____ Do you suffer with depression, mood swings, or irritability?
_____ Are you excessively sleepy?

Again, you will see from the list that symptoms of Candidisis can be similar to those associated with menopause. If you answered yes to many of the questions, you may want to consider yeast overgrowth. For more information, see the references listed at the end of this workbook including Balch's *Prescription for Nutritional Healing*, Crook's *The Yeast Connection,* Hahn's *PMS and Menopause*, or consult with a nutritional or alternative health professional familiar with Candidisis.

Menopause

Menopause refers to a single moment in time, the time of the last menstrual period. This exact time is often difficult to identify until after it has occurred. In fact, menopause is not considered to have occurred until one full year without a menstrual period. Ideally, at menopause the hormones will be in a new balance with low estrogen and progesterone levels and higher follicle stimulating hormone (FSH).

The most common test for menopause in traditional medicine is a blood test that measures FSH. The FSH hormone is responsible for stimulating the ovary to produce and egg. When no egg is released, there is no feedback mechanism to stop the production of FSH, therefore, increasing FSH to levels well above normal. When the FSH reaches a certain level, it is considered to be in the menopausal range. The test is reliable for the point in time that it is taken and does suggest that things are changing.   However, during perimenopause, levels can vary month to month, and one may still be able to become pregnant. Birth control is recommended!

Another test for menopause is a saliva test. The saliva test is more commonly used by alternative health care practitioners. The test provides information about estrogen, progesterone, and testosterone levels. At menopause these hormone levels will be decreased.

The saliva test is also useful for monitoring and comparing hormone levels when natural replacement therapies are prescribed for balancing hormones.

Postmenopause

Postmenopause refers to the stage of a women's life beginning one year after her last menstrual period. During this stage a women is no longer fertile and does not have periods. The post-menopausal stage generally lasts between 5 to 10 years and is a period of adjustment to the changed hormone levels. As in perimenopause, hormones may continue to fluctuate, and some women do experience discomforts similar to those of perimenopause. Most common discomforts are hot flashes and flushes. Some women continue to experience monthly symptoms such as bloating and breast tenderness. <u>For most women, however, all symptoms eventually stop.</u> Many women even experience what has been described as a postmenopausal zest. Postmenopausal zest is a phrase coined by anthropologist Margaret Mead. It refers to the time after menopause when women are free from periods, cramps, hormonal mood swings, and the monthly inconvenience. Women experience a renewed "zest" for life, rejuventated sex drive, and enthusiasm for new adventures or new beginnings

JOURNAL PROMPTS/ DISCUSSION QUESTIONS:
HORMONAL PHASES

- ✓ Complete the questionnaires and checklists in this section for clues to understanding your symptoms.

- ✓ What surprised you about the results of the questionnaires and checklists that you completed?

- ✓ Where are you in your hormonal transition: perimenopause, menopause, or postmenopause?

- ✓ Do you need additional information? Refer to the references and resources at the end of the workbook.

HORMONAL CHANGES AND MANAGEMENT OPTIONS

Changing hormone levels can result in various unpleasant symptoms and discomforts. Hormone replacement therapy is one option for the treatment of menopausal symptoms. There are however, alternative options as well.

Hormone Replacement Therapy

Hormone replacement therapy is commonly referred to as HRT. It is a prescription combination drug for treating the declining estrogen levels in women around the time of menopause or following a hysterectomy. HRT was originally only approved for the treatment of hot flashes and thinning bones, but it gained acceptance as a treatment for many of the conditions of aging, including heart disease.

Hormone replacement therapy (HRT) continues to be an issue for perimenopause and postmenopausal women. For years, it was believed in the traditional medical community that HRT was the magic bullet for health and well being for midlife women. Several studies questioned this premise, but it was the extensive Women's Health Initiative study conducted by National Institutes of Health that brought it to the forefront when the study determined that the risks of HRT for most women outweigh the benefits. It also raised questions about some of the actual benefits. It is now recommended that HRT should only be used to alleviate symptoms and should only be taken in the lowest effective dose for the shortest time necessary. If you are considering HRT, it is important that you know the facts.

HRT vs. ERT
HRT (Hormone Replacement Therapy) includes both estrogen and synthetic progesterone (progestin). Estrogen therapy increases one's risk of developing uterine cancer, but the addition of the progestin has been shown to reduce this risk. The down side is that the addition of progestin results in additonal risks, side effects, and in a continuation of menstrual periods. Yes, on HRT you may continue to have periods as long as you take it--even if you take it until you are 80 years old!

ERT (Estrogen only Replacement Therapy) is another prescription form of replacement therapy that was often used in the past. But because of the increased uterine cancer risk, it is now only prescribed for those who have had a hysterectomy, no longer having a uterus at risk.

Proven Benefits of Replacement Therapy (HRT and ERT)*
HRT has been shown to be effective in treating the following symptoms. These are the only conditions for which HRT has been given FDA approval:
- Vaginal dryness
- Hot flashes and night sweats
- Bone loss that contributes to osteoporosis

The benefits of using HRT are limited to the time the hormone is taken. HRT treats the symptoms of menopause. It does not "prevent" or "cure" it. It merely postpones it.   Symptoms will often return when the therapy is discontinued. In fact, bone loss rapidly increases for a period of time following the discontinuation of treatment similar to the loss that occurs with naturally occurring menopause.

There was speculation that HRT reduced the risk of heart disease, Alzheimer's disease, wrinkles, and other conditions, but there is no support for this! In fact, HRT may increase the risk of developing some of these disorders.

Possible Risks Associated with Replacement Therapy:
- Cancer of the breast
- Cancer of the uterus
- Gallbladder disease
- Abnormal blood clotting

The higher the dose the greater the risk. The number of years taking the drug is also associate with risk. The longer it is taken the greater the risk. It is now being recommended that replacement therapy should be given at the lowest possible dose necessary to reduce symptoms, and it should not be taken for more than 10 years. Not necessarily a risk but and additonal consideration is the increased medical costs for additional visits to the physician, tests, and prescriptions.

Contraindications
Women with the following conditions should not use replacement therapy because of an increased risk for complications or aggravation of symptoms.

- History of blood clots
- High blood pressure
- Unexplained vaginal bleeding
- Fibroids
- Liver disease or impairment
- Migraine headaches
- Seizure disorders
- Gallbladder disease
- Endometriosis
- History of breast cancer

Possible Side Effects of Estrogen
The following side effects may be unpleasant and are often the reasons given by women for discontinuing their use of replacement therapy.

- Nausea and vomiting
- Vaginal discharge
- Breast tenderness
- Fluid retention
- Calf cramps
- Migraine headaches

Possible Side Effects of Progestin
Progestin is the synthetic form of progesterone added to HRT to reduce the risk of uterine cancer. As you can see some of these side effects are unpleasant while others may be detrimental to your overall health.

- Decreased libido (sex drive)
- Decreased HDL (good cholesterol)
- Depressive mood
- Increased appetite
- Decreased energy level
- Weight gain
- Deepening voice
- Acne
- Increased cholesterol levels

Bioidentical Hormones
There is an increasing interest in more natural forms of hormones including bioidentical hormones. Traditional HRT estrogen is derived from pregnant horse urine and the progesterone is a synthetic form. The bioidentical hormones are milder forms of estrogen and natural progesterone rather than progestin. Some combinations even include testosterone. The doses of the hormones are balanced to achieve levels similar to those naturally occurring in the pre-menopausal body. Saliva testing is often used to determine individual's particular needs to achieve this balance. The natural hormones are said to be better and have fewer side effects because they are more like the ones produced in the human body.

These medications are prescription medications and are only available through compounding pharmacies. You may want to contact a compounding pharmacy for more information about the medications. Compounding pharmacies can also be helpful in finding a physician who is familiar with their products. Contact information for The Women's International Pharmacy is listed in the Resources Section at the end of this workbook. Check the internet or local phone books for compounding pharmacies in your area. For more information about the use of bioidentical hormones, see Suzanne Somer's books on the Reading List at the end of this workbook.

Although this method of replacement therapy is appealing, it is relatively new and there are few long-term studies of the safety of these products. Some argue that the risks of replacement are the same regardless of how the hormone is derived.

Natural Progesterone Therapy
Progesterone is the natural hormone in the body responsible for preparing the uterus for pregnancy during the childbearing years. As menopause approaches, progesterone levels fall usually faster than estrogen levels. The resulting imbalance has been identified as the possible cause of my PMS, perimenopause, and post-menopausal symptoms. Dr. John Lee and others have promoted this theory. Although prescription forms of progesterone have been used in the treatment of PMS for years, many health care professionals are cautious about Dr. Lee's impressive results with menopausal symptoms and concerns.

Administration of Natural Progesterone
Currently progesterone pills and suppositories are only available by prescription. However, non-prescription or over-the-counter progesterone creams are now available. The progesterone is absorbed through the skin. This form of administration is call transdermal. Transdermal administration has been shown to be effective. However, some of the less expensive creams contain little or no usable form of progesterone, especially those labeled as yam creams. Natural progesterone is derived from wild yam in the manufacturing process; however, it is not likely that the body will convert wild yam cream rubbed on to the skin into the useable form of progesterone. If natural progesterone is something you are interested in trying for health promotion, or as an alternative to prescription hormone therapy for dealing with menopausal symptoms, we suggest you do your research, find a reputable brand, and monitor your results. We recommend purchasing your natural progesterone cream through a health care professional or compounding pharmacy.

You may want to monitor the effectiveness of your natural progesterone treatment with saliva testing of your hormone levels. Saliva tests measure hormone levels more accurately than blood tests. Saliva test kits are available through most physicians, alternative health care practitioners, and some online labs. In addition, we recommend keeping a journal or diary of your symptoms or experiences with the cream. Some women do report problems or unpleasant side effect such as headaches, breast tenderness, or increased menstrual flow. If you experience problems, you should consult with your health care professional.

Cautions
Those who have been diagnosed with breast cancer should do more research and talk with a knowledgeable health care professional before using progesterone. The evidence is still unclear as to whether progesterone has a preventive effect or could be a possible risk.

Women taking thyroid medications should be cautious when using natural progesterone. Because progesterone has a beneficial effect on thyroid function, some women may find that they need to lower their dose of thyroid medication while using natural progesterone.

Progesterone can contribute to yeast infections. Therefore, women who have problems with yeast infections also need to be careful about using progesterone. Yeast should be controlled before starting on progesterone.

Alternative Management Options

The question about using hormone replacement therapy may be viewed as a philosophical one. Is postmenopause an unnatural state to be treated, or is postmenopause a naturally occurring stage of a woman's life, just as there are the pre-productive and reproductive stages? Women for generations have lived long, productive lives after menopause without treatment. The authors are both examples of those who made it through menopause managing our symptoms without hormone replacement.

Choosing not to use hormone replacement therapies does not mean, however, that you have to suffer risks or symptoms. Rather than looking for a magic bullet or cure-all, risks and symptoms can be treated individually often with simple measures and lifestyle choices.

The following pages identify several of the changes frequently associated with perimenopause and postmenopause. Suggestions for possible management options for each are listed. There are other supplements and approaches such as Chinese medicine or homeopathy that can also be considered. Keep in mind that the suggestions work in conjunction with a healthy diet and lifestyle. Furthermore, alternative approaches generally work slowly so they need to be given time to be effective. You may not notice the benefits for several weeks. They are not meant to be a single quick fix!

You will see that vitamin and mineral supplements are often identified as effective management options. When choosing supplements, be aware that there are differences in the quality of products. One woman was taking 900 mg of vitamin E and it was having little effect in relieving her hot flashes. When she changed to a higher-quality brand, she was able to cut back to a safer dose of 200 mg and got complete relief of her symptoms.
You want to obtain your supplements from a reliable source with reputable brands. Many health care providers now carry quality products.

Also, remember that although herbs and vitamins are natural, they can have risks, particularly if taken in large doses. Become familiar with the products and read the labels! Check for interactions with prescription medications that you may be taking. When taking supplements start slowly until you reach the optimal dose and increase only as necessary to address your symptoms. Keep track of your results. Make sure you are not double-dosing if you are taking more than one product. For example, if you are taking a multi-vitamin and decide to take vitamin E for hot flashes, check first to see how much vitamin E is in your multivitamin.   Then only add what you need to raise the dose to the desired effective dose. The fat-soluble vitamins A, D, and E are of the greatest concern because they are stored in the body and can reach harmful levels   Alternatively, excess B vitamins will be excreted through the urine. It is important, however, to recognize that taking B vitamins will and should turn your urine a "florescent" yellow color. This does not mean that you are just "flushing away the cost of the vitamin." The yellow color is the by-product of the utilization of the vitamins. It is means they are working! In fact, if your urine is not bright yellow you may need more vitamin B.

We are all unique with individual needs and responses. Therefore, we recommend:
    1) further study before using any of the approaches
    2) working with a professional who is well informed about the approaches of your choice.

Support groups are also of value for sharing additional information and evaluating experiences.

Aching Muscles and Joints and Heel Pain
Supplement suggestions
- Calcium- 500 to 1500 mg
- Magnesium- 500 to 1000 mg. Women often take calcium supplements, but in many cases magnesium is even more necessary particularly if low thyroid.
- Vitamin E- Start with 200 IU. Do not exceed 600 IU without consulting a health professional

Other suggestions
- Chiropractic adjustments

- Massage therapy
- Hydrotherapy
- Exercise, especially stretching

Anxiety and Irritability
Supplement suggestions
- Vitamin B complex- 25 mg of the B Vitamins
- Calcium- 500 to 1500 mg
- Magnesium- 500 to 1000 mg   Women often take calcium supplements, but in many cases magnesium is even more necessary
- Herbs:
  Valerian Root, Chamomile, Skull cap, Mint

Other suggestions
- Exercise- Exercise helps to get rid of excess energy, and it produces seritonin, which is the natural calming hormone
- Aromatherapy- rose and lavender
- Ibuprofen- Be sure to take ibuprofen (i.e. Motrin) and not aspirin. Ibuprofen specifically addresses the hormones, aspirin does not. Take as directed on the label. Usually 1-2 tablets every 4 to 6 hours.

Bladder Control (Incontinence)
(Loss of urine when laughing or sneezing. Or the sudden uncontrollable urge to urinate)
Supplement suggestions
- Calcium and magnesium – The bladder muscles need these minerals to be able to maintain muscle tone. 500-1000 mg

Other suggestions
- Maintain a reasonable weight
- Exercise
- Kegel exercises
- Estrogen or progesterone creams

Avoid or Limit
- Caffeine
- Alcohol
- Soft drinks

<u>Bladder Infections (Cystitis)</u>
Bladder infections are common during this period of hormonal change.
Infections may require treatment with an antibiotic. The suggestions below
are for bladder health and the prevention of infections.

Supplement suggestions
- Multivitamin including 50 mg of the major B vitamins
- Vitamin C 1000 mg daily
- Magnesium 500 – 1000 mg daily
- Calcium 500 – 1500 mg daily
- Unsweetened cranberry juice or cranberry capsules
- 8 8oz glasses of water a day. Some women find sparkling water a good alternative. Club soda is good, too. Be sure to get a brand without sodium added.

Other suggestions
- Wear cotton underwear
- Empty bladder often
- Always empty bladder after sexual intercourse- do not wait until morning

Avoid
- Alcohol
- Sugar
- Carbonated beverages
- Caffeine
- Feminine hygiene sprays
- Feminine products such as tampons or sanitary pads with fragrance

Breast Tenderness and Cysts
Supplement suggestions
- Calcium 500 to 1500 mg
- Magnesium 500 to 1000 mg   Women often take calcium supplements, but in many cases magnesium is even more necessary
- Vitamin B complex including at least 25 mg of vitamin B6
- Kelp or other source of iodine - check with your doctor before taking iodine if you have a thyroid condition
- Vitamin E 200 to 600 IU-- Start with the lower dose and work your way up if necessary.   Consult with your health care professional before taking more that 600 IU per day

Other suggestions
- Exercise helps to rid the body of excess estrogen
- Natural progesterone

Depression, Sadness
(Clinical depression should be treated by a trained health care professional)
Supplement suggestions
- Vitamin B complex 50-100 mg 3 times per day
- Vitamin C 1000 mg
- Herbs: Ginseng, St. John's Wort, Dong Quai and others have been shown to be beneficial but it is best to work with a knowlegeable professional when using herbal supplements.

Other suggestions
- Light therapy – Full spectrum light products and information are available through Sunshine Sciences at 1-800-468-1104 or www.sunshinesciences.com
- Exercise
- Improved sleep habits
- Counseling and/or talking with a friend or support group

Digestion Problems
Digestion problems often suggest the need for digestive enzymes.
Some people are just born with low levels of digestive enzymes. Others may develop a problem because of a diet high in processed, and cooked rather then fresh foods. Also, it is common for digestive enzyme levels to fall as we age. A lack of adequate digestive enzymes results in poor digestion and, therefore, poor nutrition and often digestive discomforts. Several diseases are also associated with low digestive enzyme levels including: asthma, eczema, osteoporosis, pernicious anemia, and thyroid disorders. There as several different types of digestive enzymes. Checklists associated with each are listed below.

<u>Checklist of symptoms associated with a need for pancreatic enzymes</u>
Supplement ingredients may be listed as pancreatin X4 or X5, or amylase, lipse, and protease.

_____ Inability to tolerate vegetables, especially green leafy vegetables
_____ Particles of undigested food in stool
_____ Inability to tolerate sweets, especially in the morning

_____ Gas several hours after eating

<u>Checklist of symptoms associated with a need for HCL</u>, stomach acid
*Supplement ingredients will be listed as HCL or Betaine HCL. Ox bile for
the digestion of fats may also be included.*

_____ Loss of taste for meat
_____ Need for laxatives, or diarrhea
_____ Nausea after taking vitamins
_____ Chronic yeast infections
_____ A feeling of fullness after eating or in the morning
_____ Bloating or belching after meals
_____ Gas shortly after eating
_____ Coating on tongue
_____ Bad breath
_____ Burning or itching anus
_____ Heartburn

Heartburn is often an indication of a need for more stomach acid, not
less. To test for the need for more stomach acid try taking 1
tablespoon of apple cider vinegar or lemon juice, or an HCL
supplement after eating if you are experiencing discomfort. If this
makes your discomfort less, then you need more stomach acid. If
your discomfort becomes worse, you may have too much HCL and
should not take enzyme supplements containing HCL.   Also, do not
take HCL supplements if you are taking any medicines such as aspirin
or steroids that might make the stomach bleed, without consulting
with your health care professional.

<u>Checklist of symptoms indicating the need for gallbladder supplements</u>
Supplement ingredients will include ox bile or ox bile extract.

_____ Headaches over eyes
_____ Pain between shoulder blades
_____ Bitter metallic taste in the mouth
_____ Bloating after eating fats
_____ Light colored stools
_____ Greasy foods cause discomfort

Gallbladder supplements are recommended for those who have had their gallbladders removed.

<u>Checklist of symptoms indicating a need for a supplement for the digestion of dairy products</u>
Supplement include probiotics

    _____ Lower bowel gas several hours after eating
    _____ Passing large amounts of foul smelling gas after meals
    _____ Digestive discomfort after consuming milk products
    _____ History of antibiotic use
    _____ History of corticosteroid use

Dry Eyes

Some women have difficulty wearing contacts because their eyes have become so dry.

Suggestions
- Drink plenty of liquids to stay hydrated
- Talk with your eye-care professional about the various prescription and non-prescription eye drops that are available

Avoid or limit
- Caffeine
- Antihistamines

Fatigue

Supplement suggestions
- Vitamin B complex 50 to 100 mg of the B's
- Chromium 200 mcg helps to stabilize blood sugar levels
- Drink plenty of water. Some women find sparkling water a good alternative. Club soda is good too. Be sure to get a brand without sodium added. Try a glass of water instead of coffee when feeling fatigue.
- Herbs: Ginseng

Other suggestions
- Exercise
- Have thyroid levels checked
- Be checked for anemia (Heavy menstrual blood flows may result in anemia)
- Consider Candida

- Maintain blood sugar level (eat small meals frequently)

Heart Palpitations
Supplement suggestions
- Vitamin E 200 to 600 IU-- Start with the lower dose and work your way up if necessary.   Consult with your health care professional before taking more that 600 IU per day
- Calcium 500 to 1500 mg
- Magnesium: Calcium and magnesium should be taken in a 1 to 2 ratio, in other words for every 100 mg of calcium taken, 200 mg of magnesium should be taken. Start with 250 mg calcium and 500 mg magnesium. Epsom salt foot baths are also an effective way of getting magnesium.

Other suggestions
- Drink plenty of water. Some women find sparkling water a good alternative. Club soda is good, too. Be sure to get a brand without sodium added.
- Check for allergies
- Consider Candida

Avoid or Limit
- Antihistamines
- Caffeine
- Red wine

Heartburn
Although it seems counter intuitive and contrary to popular thinking, heartburn is often a result of <u>too little</u> stomach acid rather than too much. A simple test for yourself is to take a spoonful of lemon juice or vinegar or HCL supplement after a meal or when you are experiencing symptoms. If you feel better, you probably need more stomach acid. Over the counter or prescription medications are only recommended for short term use. Because they reduce stomach acid, taking antiacids for long periods of time can lead to deficiences in the vitamins and minerals that need acid for absorption including B12, calcium, and magnesium.

Supplement suggestions
- HCL (Betaine Hydrochloride) is a digestive aid available where most vitamin supplements are sold. Take as directed.
- Zinc 30 mg daily for one month, then 15 mg daily

Avoid or limit
- Large amounts of water, especially cold water, with meals.
- Alcohol, caffeine, chocolate, citrus, mint, spicy foods, tomatoes

Heavy Menstrual Periods (The medical term is Menorrahagia)
Heavy menstrual periods may be a result of uterine fibroids, which are benign growths in the uterus, or of a medical condition known as endometriosis. See your doctor for evaluation.
Supplement suggestions
- Vitamin C with bioflavonoids (500 mg per day)
- Vitamin A   5000 IU
- Iron 25 mg to help prevent possible anemia
- Vitamin B12 200mcg

Other suggestions
- Ibuprofen- Follow the directions on the label for use, usually 1-2 tablets every 4 to 6 hours. If this is not effective, you may want to consult with a knowledgeable health care professional or resource about a different dose or different schedule. Some recommend taking ibuprofen up to a week before the period begins. Do <u>not</u> confuse ibuprofen with aspirin. Both treat pain, but they react very differently in the body. Ibuprofen is a prostaglandin hormone inhibitor, aspirin is not. Furthermore aspirin thins the blood and may make bleeding worse.
- Progesterone cream to rebalance hormones. Endometriosis and fibroids are thought to be a result of excess estrogen.
- Consult with a physician about other medical treatments. Hysterectomy is only one option. There are less traumatic options today. <u>Remember</u>, fibroids shrink naturally following menopause.

Avoid
- Alcohol- Alcohol negatively affects the blood's ability to clot, thereby increasing flow.
- Aspirin- Aspirin negatively affects the blood's ability to clot, thereby increasing flow.
- Hot baths- The heat dilates blood vessels increasing blood flow.

Hot Flashes or Night Sweats
Hot flashes and night sweats are probably the most common complaint; however, women experience them differently. Some women have nausea,

heart palpitations, or a sense of doom before the onset of a hot flash or night sweat. Others experience the hot flash as if the "heat is rising from within." Other women describe it as a flush or prickly heat sensation. A friend describes how she has a hot flash every time she dries her hair, ruining her hairdo.

Supplement suggestions
- Vitamin E   400 – 800 IU daily. Start with a low dose and add more only if needed. Do not take more than 800 IU without consulting a healthcare professional.
- Vitamin C 1000 mg
- Vitamin B complex 25-100 mg
- Blackcurrent seed oil
- Herbs: individually or in combinations including: Black cohash, Gota Kola, Dong Quai, Mother Wort, Ginseng
- Phytoestrogens (see glossary)
- Soy- There is a lot of interest in soy today. It is being promoted as an effective phytoestrogen (plant form or estrogen). However, the evidence of its health benefits is not clear.   Furthermore, it is known that soy should be avoided by some women.   Women with low thyroid, for example, should not take eat or take soy supplements! Soy, like estrogen, can interfere with thyroid function. Women with a history of breast cancer should also use soy cautiously until more is understood about its estrogenic effects.

Other suggestions
- Biofeedback
- Hypnosis
- Acupuncture, acupressure- Chinese medicine works well with the energy of hot flashes.
- Exercise- exercise helps the body eliminate excess hormones and helps to bring the hormones to normal levels
- Hard candy- A recent study suggests the hot flashes may be relate to blood sugar levels. It is important to prevent fluctuations in blood sugar levels by eating regularly and avoiding high sugar foods including soft drinks.
- Journaling- Keeping a journal gives you a sense of control
  Be sure to include the time of day of the hot flash, how it spread, how long it lasts, and what may have precipitated it. Look for patterns of behaviors you can control.

- Sometimes using <u>several</u> approaches is necessary for relieving symptoms i.e. supplements along with acupuncture or exercise.

Avoid or Limit
- Warm places, changes of temperature
- Chocolate
- Alcohol- especially red wine
- Caffeine
- Spicy or acidic foods
- White sugar
- Hydrogenated or saturated fats
- Dairy products

Memory Loss

The memory loss associated with menopause can be frightening and frustrating, but is usually only temporary. Furthermore, although some changes in memory and quick recall are associated with aging, it is not necessarily a predictor of Alzheimer's disease.

Supplement suggestions
- Vitamin B complex   25-100 mg
- Rescue remedy- a homeopathic remedy

Other suggestions
- Reduce stress
- Accept the fact that slower recall does not mean memory loss.
- Mental confusion and memory problems resulting from hormone imbalance <u>do</u> improve after menopause.
- Check for other health problems such as thyroid, Candida, vitamin deficiencies, or medication side effects.

Sleeplessness

Sleeplessness is a common and frustrating complaint of menopausal women. Often the sleeplessness is a result of other midlife issues such as stress or hot flashes, and then the sleeplessness contributes to fatigue and mental confusion. It is a vicious cycle.

Supplement suggestions
- Calcium 500-1500 mg- especially if you have trouble <u>getting to sleep</u>
- Magnesium 500-1000 mg -if you can get to sleep but <u>wake up frequently</u>

- Melatonin
- Herbs: Chamomile tea, Valerian root, or combinations

Other suggestions
- Exercise
- Relaxation techniques such as deep breathing, yoga, meditation
- Acupuncture
- Massage
- Waking up between 3:00 and 4:00AM may be a result of falling blood sugar levels. Eating a low carbohydrate snack such as cheese or nuts before bed can be helpful in preventing the blood sugar level from falling. Eating something when you wake up during the night, such as a whole-wheat cracker or a glass of orange juice, can be helpful in raising the blood sugar level and help get you back to sleep.

Vaginal Dryness, Difficulty With Intercourse

As hormone levels change, there is less lubrication of the vagina often making intercourse painful or uncomfortable.

Supplement suggestions
- Vitamin E – orally, or as a cream, or vaginal suppository
- Omega 3 fatty acids - taken as a supplement or from a diet that includes fish atleast 2 times a week
- Vitamin B complex
- Herbs such as black cohash and licorice
- Water- 8 8oz cups a day to keep hydrated

Other suggestions
- "Use it or lose it" Frequent intercourse helps to keep the tissues lubricated
- Warm baths before intercourse
- More or longer foreplay may be necessary to stimulate the natural lubrication
- Lubricating jelly such KY jelly or other water based product (NOT petroleum jelly)
- Wear cotton-crotch underwear
- Exercise increases blood flow to the pelvic area
- Kegel exercises (see glossary)

Avoid
- Deodorant soaps can be irritating

- Hygiene sprays can be irritating
- Antihistamines contribute to dryness
- Caffeine contributes to dryness
- Alcohol affects vaginal health

<u>Vaginal Infections</u>

Vaginal infections are common during periods of hormonal change. Infections may need to be treated with a prescription or over-the-counter antibiotic. The suggestions below are for maintaining a healthy vagina for the prevention of infection.

Supplement suggestions
- Vitamin B complex   50 – 100 mg daily
- Vitamin C 1000 mg daily
- Probiotics- tablets or capsules are the best source. Look for quality supplements that supply billions of live microorganisms. Yogurt is often recommended as a source of probiotics, however, dairy products and the sugars in yogurt may actually contribute to problem. Also, some of the less expensive brands of yogurt do not contain any active acidophilus culture. Do not rely on yogurt as a source of probiotics when you have an infection.

Other suggestions
- Wear cotton-crotch underwear
- Take additional probiotic when taking antibiotics for any reason

Avoid
- Hygiene spray
- Douching
- Sugar
- *Alcohol*

Summary

In reviewing the management suggestions, you will see that there are some recurring themes. These include <u>physical exercise, Kegel exercises (see glossary), vitamin and mineral supplements--especially the B's-- and calcium and magnesium, reducing stress, and limiting sugar, alcohol, and caffeine intake.</u>

Exercise has been identified as one of the best things you can do for yourself. If in fact there is a <u>"magic bullet," it is probably exercise</u>. It not only adds years to your life, but it improves the quality of life. Even a gentle stroll for half an hour a day has been shown to be beneficial. Walking with friends can be great. Not only are you getting a workout, but you are also enjoying the benefits of a support group. If walking does not appeal to you, how about ballroom dancing, tap dancing, or even just adding additional steps to your day by parking in the farthest parking place rather than the nearest at the mall or grocery store?

Supplements are also important. There is increasing evidence of their value for most everyone. It is difficult to meet our daily requirements through our diet alone with our busy life styles, dieting, and food preferences. A good quality multivitamin/ mineral supplement makes it easier than taking handfuls of individual supplements. Furthermore, vitamins and minerals work best in conjunction with each other. When choosing supplements read the labels and look for optimal levels (ODA), rather than just RDA (recommended daily allowance). The RDA's are the minimal levels established by the FDA to prevent deficiency diseases. Higher levels are valuable in achieving health and reducing symptoms. To achieve the higher levels, a typical multivitamin/mineral supplement dose of 3-6 tablets a day will be required.

We recommend that you start slowly, taking just one or two tablets a day for a few days to see how you react. Then add another tablet each day working up to the desired number of tablets a day. If you experience stomach discomfort try taking your supplements with meals. Taking additional HCL can also be helpful if you have trouble digesting vitamins and minerals.

General recommendations for daily NUTRITIONAL SUPPLEMENTATION FOR MIDLIFE WOMEN

Vitamin A (as beta carotene)--5000 IU
Vitamin D--400 IU
Vitamin E--200 IU
Vitamin B1--50-100 mg
Vitamin B2---15-50 mg
Vitamin B3(niacin)--15-50 mg
Vitamin B5(pantothenic acid)-------------------------------------50-100 mg
Vitamin B6--50-100 mg
Vitamin B12---200 mcg
Vitamin C---1000 mg
Bioflavonoids---800 mg
Pantothenic acid--50 mg
Choline--50 mg
Inositol--50 mg
PABA (para-aminobenzoic acid)--------------------------------------50 mg
Folic acid--400 mg
Calcium---1200 mg
Magnesium*--750 mg
    *Magnesium levels should be 2 to 1 ratio with calcium if experiencing
    symptoms such as PMS, heart palpations, low thyroid, anxiety i.e. 500
    mg of magnesium, 250 mg of calcium.*
Iodine---150 mcg
Iron* ---25 mg
    *Iron supplements should be taken with caution or not at all
    after menopause when there is no longer blood loss with periods.*
Copper---2 mg
Zinc--35 mg
Manganese---3-10 mg
Potassium---100 mg
Selenium---25-100 mcg
Chromium--150 mcg
Boron---3 mg

From: Balch, Phyllis A. <u>Prescription for Nutritional Healing. 5th editon</u>. New York: Penguin Group. 2010.

This is a long list. You may choose to take a daily multivitamin/mineral supplement with everything in it. But remember, to get these optimal levels the daily dose will be three to six tablets. Alternatively, you can use this list as a reference and customize your own plan based on you own particular symptoms and needs. For example, if you eat a lot of dairy products you may not need to take additional calcium, or if you have trouble sleeping through the night, you may want to take additional magnesium. Talking with a nutritionist or naturopathy physician would be helpful in determining your particular needs.

JOURNAL PROMPTS/ DISCUSSION QUESTIONS:
HORMONE CHANGES AND MANAGEMENT OPTIONS

✓ What is your philosophical position on aging and changing hormone levels? Is it a natural state or one to be treated?

✓ What experience have you or your friends had with HRT or ERT? Was it positive or negative?

✓ It is important "know" your own body. Pay attention to what you are feeling and when. What are your physical concerns?
When do they occur? Monthly? Daily? After eating certain foods or doing certain activities?

✓ How do emotional factors affect your symptoms; i.e. did you feel worse after a disagreement with your child or spouse?

✓ What in your medical history may be a factor in your symptoms, i.e. past yeast infections?

✓ Review the list of changes and management options. Are there some options you would like to try? Do additional research on them.

    o When trying options be sure to evaluate how they are working. What works for you; what doesn't? For example, what supplements have you tried or are you trying? Write down the amounts taken, the brand, and the dates used. Do they make a difference?

IMPORTANT MIDLIFE HEALTH ISSUES

Cardiovascular Disease

Cardiovascular disease is a real concern for postmenopausal women. After menopause a women's risk of heart disease approaches that of men. However, traditionally physicians have viewed heart disease as a disease of men. Women's symptoms have been more likely attributed to non-cardiac causes than men's. Women have been less likely to be referred for cardiac catheterization or bypass surgery than men. Women's treatments typically start later in the course of their disease, therefore increasing their risk of death. This disparity in care is changing, but slowly.

There is also increasing understanding that heart disease in women and men is different. Women's symptoms are often different than men's. Women are less likely to have the excruciating pain down the left arm, but women are more likely to have anxiety, shortness of breath, or jaw pain. Furthermore, obstructions in men are commonly in the large heart vessels, but in women the obstructions may more likely be in smaller vessels. Consequently, the standard tests such as the treadmill stress test or angiograms may not be effective in diagnosing women. Therefore, it is important for women to be informed about cardiovascular disease and be prepared to be their own advocates for appropriate diagnosis and treatment!

Myths about Heart Disease:
- *Heart disease is for men and cancer is for women*

- *Heart disease is only of concern for old people*

- *Heart disease doesn't affect women who are physically fit*

Facts about Heart Disease:
- *Cardiovascular disease (heart attack or stroke) is the leading cause of death in women over 50 years of age.*

- *Women's symptoms of a heart attack may be different from those of men. Women are less likely to experience pain in the left arm but will more likely have nausea, anxiety, shortness of breath, unusual weakness or fatigue.*

- *HRT has <u>not</u> been shown to protect women from cardiovascular disease. It may, in fact, contribute to strokes.*

Risk Factors
The following is a list of factors that increase your risk of developing heart disease.
- Menopause before the age of 45 years
- A strong family history of cardiovascular disease
- Excessive body fat around you waist or upper body
- Smoking
- A sedentary lifestyle
- Poor diet
- High blood pressure
- Diabetes
- Magnesium deficiency

Prevention
The following are some options for reducing your risks of developing or suffering with heart disease.

Exercise is very important. Even a casual walk for 30 minutes a day is helpful.

Supplements
- Vitamin A 5000 IU
- Vitamin E 400-800 IU
- Magnesium 500 mg (more if a coffee and/or alcohol drinker)

Limit
- Smoking
- Alcohol
- Iron supplements after menopause

Summary
Women need take responsibility for their own cardiovascular health. First, women need to be aware of the risks and recognize that there are some simple life style choices that can effectively reduce those risks. Secondly, women need to be prepared to be their own advocate in the health care delivery system demanding appropriate concern, testing, and treatment.

Osteoporosis

One of the major concerns for menopausal women is osteoporosis. Osteoporosis is the thinning of the bones that may result in fractures. This focus on osteoporosis has only recently become a major concern. In the past, osteoporosis was defined as a disease where bones fracture easily as a result of little impact because they have become thin, brittle, and weak. It was somewhat uncommon and could occur at any age. Today osteoporosis has come to mean a condition of low mineral density <u>without</u> necessarily clear evidence of increased risk of fracture! Much of the new interest in this condition has been a result of advertising by the pharmaceutical and dairy industries and the development of new tools for measuring bone density.

Myths about Osteoporosis:
- *All women over the age of 50 are at risk for osteoporosis (brittle bones).*

- *Osteoporosis is the cause of bone fractures in the elderly.*

- *Women die of osteoporosis.*

- *The measurement of bone density is a reliable measure of risk for fracture.*

- *High calcium and dairy intake prevents osteoporosis.*

Facts about Osteoporosis:
- *Only about 20% of white and Asian women, 10% of Hispanic women, and 5% of African- American women age 50 or older are believed to have osteoporosis according to the National Osteoporosis Foundation.*

- *Bone loss accelerates at menopause at the rate of 2% per year for up to 7 years. After the body adjusts to its new hormone levels, the bone loss is equal to that of a man the same age.*

- *The best prevention for osteoporosis is to be active and have an adequate intake of calcium as a teenager when bones are still forming. The more bone mass you have to start with, the more you can afford to lose. This is important for our teenage daughters. They need to be active, take their calcium, and limit the number of soft drinks they consume. Soft drinks rob the body of calcium. The phosphates in carbonated soft drinks cause the elimination of calcium from the body and bones.*

- *Women can continue to build new bone mass even after menopause.*

- *Hormone replacement therapy does not prevent bone loss. It only postpones it until you stop taking the hormones. Then the bone loss accelerates for the 7-year period as the body adjusts to the new hormone levels, as with natural menopause.*

- *People do not die of osteoporosis. They die or suffer from the complications of resulting fractures. Prevention of fractures is critical.*

- *Hip fractures are the leading cause of admission to nursing homes. However, most women who suffer hip fractures are over the age of 85 and are unwell.*

- *The dairy and pharmaceutical industries are responsible for much of our increased awareness of osteoporosis.*

- *Dark green vegetables such as broccoli and greens are better sources of calcium than milk.*

- *Weight-bearing exercise has been shown to increase bone mass. In fact, weight-bearing exercise has been shown to be more beneficial than some of the osteoporosis drugs on the market.*

Risk Factors
The following are the risk factors that have been identified for developing brittle bones.
- Fair complexion
- Thin and small bones
- Early menopause naturally (younger than age 45)
- Ovaries removed without replacement hormone therapy
- Family history of osteoporosis
- No pregnancies
- Smoking
- Lack of regular physical activity
- Lack of regular physical activity as a child or teen when most bone mass is established

- High intake of alcohol, coffee, tea, or cola (These rob the body of the necessary nutrients for bone building)
- Low dietary calcium intake
- Regular use of cortisone, anti-seizure medications, anticoagulants, or antibiotics
- Liver or kidney disease, digestive disorder, or over-active thyroid
- Ancestors from England, Ireland, Scotland, Northern Europe, or Asia

Prevention

There are several options for preventing or limiting the risk of developing brittle bones. These include lifestyle choices and supplements, as well as medical options.

Hormone Replacement

Estrogen- Estrogen helps to maintain bone mass. It does not increase bone mass. The benefits of the estrogen are limited to the time it is taken. If for example you take HRT or ERT from age 50 to 60, then you will begin a period of rapid bone loss at age 60 rather than 50.

Progesterone- There is some evidence that natural progesterone may be effective in helping to build new bone mass. However, progestin, the synthetic form of progesterone that is added to HRT to lower the risk of uterine cancer, does not have an effect on the bones.

Prescription Drugs

There are new drugs coming on the market all of the time. You should talk with your health care provider if you think this is something for you. Remember they all have risks, as well as, benefits. It is important to assess your risk for fracture when weighing the risks and benefits of the drug. Some of the drugs on the market have been shown to increase bone density but not bone strength making bones <u>more</u> not less likely to fracture. In fact, the NWHN (National Women's Health Network) believes that "using osteopenia (bone density lower than normal) as a justification to start medication treatment is dangerous- the benefit of treating osteorosis preventatively almost never outweights the risks that treatments pose."

Supplements
- Calcium 1500 mg *
- Magnesium 500 mg

- Zinc 15 mg
- Boron 3 mg
- Vitamin D 400 IU

*Calcium is not enough. The other minerals are equally important and in many cases more important. We often get significant amounts of calcium in our diets if we eat dairy and vegetables. Magnesium and boron are less available. Supplements that contain a combination of the minerals necessary for bone building are available. *Osteo B* by Biotics Research is a good one.

Other options
Exercise- Weight-bearing exercise, exercises such as running or walking where you are supporting your own weight has been shown to increase bone mass. In fact, weight-bearing exercise has been shown to be more beneficial than some of the osteoporosis drugs on the market for all ages. Exercise for flexibility and balance is also important for preventing falls.

Accident prevention measures- Remember, fractures usually are a result of falls; therefore it is the falls that need to be prevented. Accident proof the home. Eliminate loose cords, loose throw rugs, and slippery surfaces. Be aware of medication side effects that can cause dizziness or confusion that may result in falls.

Good news about weight gain in menopause. It has been suggested that extra fat especially in the hip area protects against fractures.

Avoid or Limit:
The following should be avoided or limited because of their negative effect on calcium levels. These behaviors and substances decrease calcium levels by increasing calcium excretion from the body or decreasing absorption.
- Smoking
- Protein and red meat
- Alcohol
- Diuretics
- Caffeine
- Sugar
- Soft drinks
- Anti-heartburn medications

Testing
Bone density testing is becoming increasing popular to determine if bones
are thinning. The test measures bone density, not fracture risk! There are
many factors in addition to aging that contribute to fracture risk.
If you are considering being tested, you should be clear as to why you are
having the test and what you will do with the results. Medical experts now
recommend that women wait until age 65 to be screened for osteoporosis.
Remember <u>testing only gives a measurement; it is not a preventative
treatment</u>!

- Are you looking for a baseline?
- Are you willing to take medications if recommended?
- Are looking for that incentive you need to start a workout program or
  vitamin/mineral regime?

If you have the test, it is also important that you have an understanding of
your results. Be sure and talk to you health care professional to determine
what your test result numbers mean for you.

- Are your numbers high or low compared to the general population,
  young women, or in comparison to other women your age?
  Remember, some bone loss is expected as we age.
- Have your numbers changed significantly? Remember, rate of bone
  loss accelerates at menopause at the rate of 2% per year for up to 7
  years. But, after the body adjusts to its new hormone levels, the bone
  loss is equal to that of a man the same age.

Breast Cancer

It is almost impossible to enter into a discussion with a group of midlife women, and not find at least one person whose life has been touched by breast cancer: either her own, or that of a relative or a friend. Women used to hide this "disease" out of fear or shame or embarrassment. Today, women are much more willing to discuss how this dreaded "C" word has impacted their lives. More and more women have insurance that pays for annual mammograms. New digital mammography units are able to detect breast cancer with fewer and fewer "false positives" that result in unnecessary biopsies.

New treatments are being developed every year. Some women choose to have a lumpectomy. Others who have done genetic testing, may decide to have a mastectomy to prevent breast cancer. Treatment options range from chemotherapy and radiation to drugs like Tamoxifen. All have their own long-range side effects, and each woman must do her own research to determine which course of treatment will work best for her given her family history, the progression of the disease, and her own comfort levels.

Unfortunately now that managed care dominates the health care industry, all of us need to be our own researchers and advocates when it comes to the issue of breast cancer.

Myths of Breast Cancer:
- *If I have no family history of breast cancer, I can't get breast cancer.*

- *If I breast fed my children, I can't get breast cancer.*

- *If I am under age 50, I can't get breast cancer.*

- *If I get a mastectomy, I can prevent breast cancer or a reoccurrence of breast cancer.*

- *If I never take HRT, I won't get breast cancer.*

- *If I can't feel a lump, I don't have breast cancer.*

- *I exercise and keep my weight under control, so I won't get breast cancer.*

Facts of Breast Cancer: (Breastcancer.org)
- *Besides skin cancer, breast cancer is the most commonly diagnosed cancer among American women About 1 in 8 U.S. women (about 12.4%) will develop invasive breast cancer over the course of her lifetime.*

- *Breast cancer incidence rates in the U.S. began decreasing in the year 2000, after increasing for the previous two decades. One theory is that this decrease was partially due to the reduced use of hormone replacement therapy (HRT) by women.*

- *Death rates have been decreasing since 1989. Women under 50 have experienced larger decreases. These decreases are thought to be the result of treatment advances, earlier detection through screening, and increased awareness.*

- *About 5-10% of breast cancers can be linked to gene mutations (abnormal changes) inherited from one's mother or father.*

- *There can be a rich, full life after breast cancer. Even after treatment one can feel "normal again." One can regain strength, energy, vitality, and zest for life.*

Risk factors
- Smoking- particularly if taking estrogen
- Estrogen- as in birth control or HRT
- Genetic predisposition, family history
- Alcohol use

Prevention

Although monthly breast examination and yearly mammograms will not prevent breast cancer they may identify cancer in its earliest stage for early intervention and better outcome.

Mammograms

There has been a lot of controversy about mammograms in the news lately. Women are not sure when to start getting mammograms. Here are the guidelines from the American Cancer Society:
- Women ages 40 to 44 should have the choice to start annual breast cancer screening with mammograms (x-rays of the breast) if they wish to do so.

- Women age 45 to 54 should get mammograms every year.

- Women 55 and older should switch to mammograms every 2 years, or can continue yearly screening.

- Screening should continue as long as a woman is in good health and is expected to live 10 more years or longer.

-

- All women should be familiar with the known benefits, limitations, and potential harms linked to breast cancer screening.

Women should also know how their breasts normally look and feel and report any breast changes to a health care provider right away.

Genetic Testing

Many women with a family history of breast cancer, think about having genetic testing done. Of course, that must be a decision that each woman makes for herself. However, here are some things to consider:

- Genetic testing is quite expensive and may not be covered by your insurance.

- Once you have the genetic testing done, if it turns out that you do have the genetic mutation markers for breast cancer, you will be classified by health care insurance providers as having a "pre-existing condition."

- Many women, who have the genetic mutation marker for a disease, may never develop the disease. New research is being done daily about what other factors "turn on and off" specific genes.

- Once you have any kind of test done, you must be prepared to deal with the test results if they are negative. For breast cancer, this not only involves much anxiety and fear, but many breast doctors will recommend a single or double mastectomy. Sometimes they will also want to remove the ovaries. These decisions have life-altering consequences.

Management with Treatment

Galen Magee (Jayne's son, a fashion designer) designs beautiful robes that make women feel beautiful while they are undergoing treatment for breast cancer. The robes can be purchased at: www.jaynesrobe.com. For every robe purchased, one robe is given away to a woman who is undergoing treatment for breast cancer, but cannot afford to buy a robe for herself.

New research is ongoing about the positive effects of exercise in mitigating some of the worst side effects of chemotherapy such as fatigue, nausea, and pain.

Women have also found that yoga and meditation, prayer, and journaling help them to cope better as they struggle to find relief from physical, emotional and mental pain during cancer treatments.

JOURNAL PROMPTS/ DISCUSSION QUESTIONS:
IMPORTANT MIDLIFE HEALTH ISSUES

- ✓ What are your risk factors for developing heart disease?

- ✓ What are you doing or can you do to reduce or minimize your risks?

- ✓ What are your risk factors for developing osteoporosis?

- ✓ What are you doing or can you do to reduce your risk?

- ✓ If you are considering having a bone density test, be sure to answer the questions about why you are having it done:
  Are you looking for a baseline?
  Are you willing to take medications if recommended?
  Are looking for that incentive you need to start a workout program or vitamin/mineral regime?

- ✓ If you have had a bone density test, what did your results mean for you?

- ✓ What are your risk factors for developing breast cancer? Do you get regular mammograms? If not, why not?

SECTION TWO:
<u>Psychological and Emotional Concerns of Midlife</u>

MIDLIFE STRESSORS

Midlife is a time of stress for both men and women. More of life's stressful events occur during midlife than during any other one period of time. It is also during midlife that we begin to face or our own mortality. We start asking, "Is this all there is?" "Am I running out of time?" Children are leaving home; aging parents are moving in or needing care. These are difficult situations when accompanying emotions reactions. We may experience this stress as a Blue Funk. A period of feeling down or off a little.

Life Changes
In a famous study done in 1967 but still recognized as valid, Drs. Thomas H. Holmes and Richard H. Rahe identified a list of 43 major life stressors. Each event was assigned a scale of impact value. The list includes event such as: death of a spouse (100 points), divorce (73 points), marital separation (65 points), death of a close family member (63 points), personal injury or illness (53 points), retirement (45 points), sexual difficulties (39 points), death of a close friend (37 points), child leaving home (29 points), and spouse beginning or leaving work (26 points). *See the next page for the complete questionnaire.*

The total score is a measure of risk for illness. Because of the negative effects stress has on the body, the higher the score, the higher the risk of becoming ill. The illness can range from the flu to something more serious such as depression.   As you can see from the list many of life's most stressful events typically occur in midlife. Is it any wonder we often experience illness and depression in midlife?

There is good news. Stress related illness is not inevitable! The single factor that the sociologists found to be effective in keeping us well is social support. Those with the most social support have the lowest risk of developing illness. Social support may come from family, friends or support groups.

HOLMES AND RAHE LIFE CHANGE INDEX
Thomas H. Holmes and Richard H. Rahe

If an event has been true for you in the past year or will occur in the near future, copy the number in the left column over to the right column. Then total the points.

Event	Scale of impact	Score
Death of a spouse*	100	_____
Divorce	73	_____
Marital separation	65	_____
Jail term	63	_____
Death of a close family member*	63	_____
Personal injury or illness*	53	_____
Marriage	50	_____
Fired at work	47	_____
Marital reconciliation	45	_____
Retirement*	45	_____
Change in health of a family member*	44	_____
Pregnancy	40	_____
Sexual difficulties*	39	_____
Gain of a new family member	39	_____
Business readjustment	39	_____
Change in financial status	38	_____
Death of a close friend*	37	_____
Change to a different line of work	36	_____
Change in the number of arguments with spouse	35	_____
Mortgage over $20,000	31	_____
Foreclosure of mortgage or loan	30	_____
Change in responsibilities at work	29	_____
Son or daughter leaving home*	29	_____
Trouble with in-laws	29	_____
Outstanding personal achievement	28	_____
Spouse begins or stops work*	26	_____
Beginning or end school	26	_____
Change in living conditions	25	_____
Revision of personal habits	24	_____
Trouble with your boss	23	_____
Change in work hours or conditions	20	_____
Change in residence	20	_____
Change in schools	20	_____

Change in recreation	19	_____
Change in church activities	19	_____
Change in social activities	18	_____
Mortgage or loan less than $20,000	17	_____
Change in sleeping habits	16	_____
Change in the number of family get togethers*	15	_____
Change in eating habits	15	_____
Vacation	13	_____
Christmas (if approaching)	12	_____
Minor violation of the law	11	_____

Your score is an indication of your risk for developing an illness, physical or mental in the next 12 months.

To determine your score, add up the values in the right column.
A score ranging from 0 to 149 has a risk factor of 30%
A score ranging from 150 to 299 has a risk factor of 50%
A score of 300 or more has a risk factor of 80%

   * events associated with midlife

Midlife Blue Funk
Accompanying the midlife, stressful life changes, there are often mood changes, a malaise, and thoughts that we identify as the Blue Funk. Do any of these feelings sound familiar?

- I don't seem to have the energy I had when I was younger.
- I often feel draggy or listless.
- I sometimes feel depressed for no apparent reason.
- My old interests don't seem important any more, and sometimes I can't even remember what they were.
- I'm finding my everyday duties and activities boring or oppressive.
- I seem to overreact to even small irritations.
- I find myself obsessively worrying about even little things.
- Sometimes I feel like I am going crazy.
- I find it difficult to make a decision and wish others would make them for me.
- I seem to be having trouble remembering things, and I am bothered by it.
- Sometimes I have trouble thinking clearly or staying focused.
- I often feel that I am useless or a failure.
- I feel that everyone takes advantage of me.
- Sometimes I get a foreboding feeling for no apparent reason.
- I often wish I could run away and escape my present situation.
- My interest in sex has decreased.
- At times I have romantic notions or daydreams about someone other than my partner.
- I find myself enjoying romantic novels or soap operas as an escape.
- I have been thinking a lot about "what might have been."
- I am spending a lot of time thinking about who I am and what I have become.
- I've been wondering, "When is it my turn?"
- I've been asking myself, "Is this all there is!"

The feelings identified with the Blue Funk may be confusing and maybe even a little frightening to you. We include the checklist here so you will know that you are not alone in having these feelings. You are not going crazy or losing your mind. As our friend Karen said, "It is reassuring to know that the feelings I am experiencing are normal because they are not typical for me." <u>The Blue Funk is not abnormal and will pass in time.</u> If these feelings linger, however, or you find yourself so preoccupied that you are unable to function normally, you may want to seek processional help.

Journal Prompts/ Discussion Questions:

MIDLIFE STRESSORS

- ✓ Complete the Holmes and Rahe checklist to determine your level of stress or distress.

- ✓ What methods or strategies do you use to reduce the stress levels in your life?

- ✓ In our busy lives and transient society, we often find ourselves alone. Do you have a source of social support? How can you develop or expand your social network? How about a walking group for social support and exercise?

- ✓ Are you experiencing the Blue Funk? Are you aware of others who are having similar thoughts and feelings?

- ✓ What methods or strategies might you use to cope with the Blue Funk?

MIDLIFE AS A GRIEF PROCESS

Losses
Many of the life changes identified by Holmes and Rahe involve losses. Many of these losses, such as the loss of parents and friends or the loss of a job, and facing our own mortality can be associated with midlife for both men and women. Women may experience additional losses such as the loss of youth and beauty, the loss of sense of self, and a changing role as a mother.

As women age, many must confront the loss of youth and beauty associated with fairytales like *Cinderella* and *Sleeping Beauty*. Our society values beauty, and beauty is associated with youth. Therefore, as a woman loses her youth she may feel that she has also lost her value as well, like the Wicked Stepmother in *Snow White*.

Midlife is also a time of loss of self. Having spent years putting their own desires aside and instead putting the desires of their husband's, their children's, and/or their career's first, midlife women may feel that they have lost themselves. We hear women lamenting that they no longer even know their own likes and dislikes. They have forgotten their former passions or have failed to develop new ones. After "speaking" to please others for so many years midlife women have lost their "own voice."

Furthermore, many women's dreams and identity as a woman are associated with being a mother. Now that the children are leaving home and their fertility is gone, many women struggle with the "dreaded" Empty Nest syndrome. Who am I now if I am not a mother? On a positive note, more current research has shown that depression is not inevitable when children leave home. In fact, many women today actually look forward to it. However, no matter how a woman feels about it, it is still a loss, an adjustment. Much of our "busyness" is gone. Have you ever looked back over your old calenders and wondered how you did it all?

Of course, there are the women who have never had children. They, too, are thinking, "Is this all there is?" Maybe I should have had children. Is it too late?"

 The following are losses that many women experience at midlife:

- Perceived loss of our physical beauty
- Perceived loss of our femininity
- Loss of fertility
- Loss of our energy and enthusiasm
- Loss of ourselves, our "Voices"
- Loss of our goals and dreams
- Loss of our expectations: what we thought we were going to do or be
- Loss of breasts to cancer
- Loss of spouse to death or divorce
- Loss of parents, friends, family members
- Loss of the Glass Slipper: our myths and fairy tale endings of living "happily ever after."

These losses must be grieved before we can move forward. The Midlife Grieving Process is comprised of the following stages: denial, anger, acceptance, and reinvention.

Grief is a process that takes time.   We must be cautious not to make rash decisions during this time period. Running away from or divorcing the "loser" may seem like the answer now, but it may not be the best solution in the long run.   The best way to process midlife as a Grief Process is to slow down and allow it to happen.

Journal Prompts / Discussion Questions:
MIDLIFE AS A GREIF PROCESS- LOSSES

- ✓ Make a list of your losses. What are you grieving?

- ✓ How do you express your grief?

- ✓ Which of your losses are specific to being a woman in the 21st century?

- ✓ Which of your losses are specific to menopause?

- ✓ Which of your losses are specific to aging?

Stage One: Denial

The first stage of grief is denial. When a loss occurs, we first try to protect ourselves from the pain by denying the loss. Women may try to deny the loss of youth and beauty with cosmetics, diets, exercise, or plastic surgery. Other ways of denying the changes of midlife include dating younger men, refusing to talk about menopause, or searching for a "magic bullet" that will make us feel the same way that we have always felt. A late in life baby can also be a form of an attempt to postpone an end to mothering. The media also denies the reality of midlife either by making women look younger than they actually are on TV and in the movies or by just not using actresses who are over fifty. Have you ever noticed that older men in the movies are typically in love with much younger women?

Another way to deny the grief of midlife losses is to numb ourselves with alcohol, food, excessive exercising, workaholism, busyness, shopping, or drugs. While all of those things may temporarily dull the pain of the losses, eventually they must be dealt with if we want to enjoy a healthy, vibrant, and productive life after fifty. When the denial no longer works, the next stage is anger.

Journal Prompts/ Discussion Questions:
MIDLIFE AS A GREIF PROCESS- STAGE 1: DENIAL

- ✓ Which of your losses or changes are you denying?

- ✓ Make a list of the ways you or women you know are denying the changes of midlife.

Stage Two: Anger

Anger follows denial after loss. The anger of grief can be specific to the loss, such as anger toward someone who has taken something from you, but it can also become generalized. If the anger becomes pervasive, it can affect every area of our lives. In discussion groups with midlife women, the following issues of anger were identified:

- Is this all there is?
- Life isn't fair.
- I'm sick of trying to be a good girl and doing the right thing.
- I thought if I just did it all I would have it all.
- I thought by now I wouldn't have any money worries. What happened?
- I wish that I had never gotten married.
- I am sorry that I never married.
- I am sorry that never had children.
- I'm mad at the medical industry for treating my menopause as if it is a disease.
- I'm tired of never being valued by society for what I do.
- I hate being judged because I'm no longer young and beautiful.
- I'm angry with my body because I can no longer control it.
- I don't have time to deal with menopause.
- I've spent my whole life doing things other people wanted me to do. I gave up my dreams for my family and/or career. When is it My Turn?
- I don't want to get sick and die.
- I am so stressed dealing with children, my job, and elderly parents.
- I am angry that my parents are sick and are dying.

Women often feel that it is not okay to be angry. However, if the anger of midlife is not recognized and expressed it will either develop into rage, or be suppressed resulting in self-blame and depression. Neither of these outcomes is healthy. How many women do you know who are currently taking anti-depressants for midlife depression? We have other choices.

Women are allowed to be angry! It doesn't mean you have to act on it. It is just important that you recognize it and allow yourself to feel it. Sometimes it may be helpful to yell out loud or beat on a pillow. One friend, Loretta, finds "rock throwing" an effective technique for getting out anger. Loretta suggests going out into your yard, collecting rocks of various sizes and shapes each representing a different source of anger, and throwing them as hard and as far as possible. It helps to dispel the energy of the anger that can become destructive.

Journal Prompt/ Discussion Questions
MIDLIFE AS A GREIF PROCESS- STAGE 2: ANGER

- ✓ What might you be angry about?

- ✓ What have your disappointments been?

- ✓ Do you feel that life has treated you fairly? Are you living "happily ever after"? If not, what happened to your fairytale ending?

- ✓ Do you allow yourself to feel anger?

- ✓ How do you express your anger?

- ✓ Are there healthier ways to express your anger? If so, what might some of those be?

Stage Three: Acceptance
After recognizing our losses, and allowing ourselves to feel angry, we need to move on to acceptance. Yes, in fact, we are getting older. Life isn't always fair, no matter how good we have been or how much we plan. Our hair is turning gray, and we are getting thicker around the middle. The children do grow up. All of our dreams may not have come true.

Acceptance does not necessarily mean we have to like these losses, but we do need to recognize that denying or ruminating won't change things. No more "would have," "could have," or "should have's." We must move forward and remember getting older isn't all bad. Acceptance means that we have quit fighting the changes that midlife and menopause bring. Acceptance involves the recognition that many midlife and menopausal changes are positive, not negative.

Facts about Acceptance:
- We can't control everything.
- Life isn't perfect or fair.
- Midlife is just another stage of life.
- Our roles are changing.
- Menopause is a natural, normal part of life—not a "disease."
- Hot flashes cleanse the body of impurities, so we stay healthier.
- No more messy periods!!!
- Studies show that women are healthier after menopause.
- Old ladies don't have to follow the rules anymore. They can say what they really think and get away with it!
- We are full of wisdom.
- We can challenge our creativity and intellect: question everything and think for ourselves.
- We become less worried about what others may think of us. More self-acceptance.
- We have postmenopausal zest! We are free to reinvent ourselves. It is finally our turn—we have permission to put ourselves first.

Journal Prompts/ Discussion Questions
MIDLIFE AS A GREIF PROCESS- STAGE 3: ACCEPTANCE

- ✓ What do you need to learn to accept in midlife?

- ✓ Which of the positive changes about getting older most resonate with you?

- ✓ What are some other good things that you can think of about getting older?

Stage Four: Reinvestment
After recognizing our losses, being angry about them, and finally accepting our new stage in life it is time for reinvesting our energy and reinventing ourselves if necessary for the next stage of our life. It is a time of opportunity. Typically women spend the early stages of their lives pleasing and taking care of others. This new stage is what has been referred to as "my time." My time is a time for pleasing and taking care of ourselves, a time for self fulfillment. At midlife there is a reawakening for women like that of the fairy tale princesses when kissed by the princes. However, in contrast to the myths, we have the power to reawaken ourselves.

This stage involves looking at every area of our lives and then deciding what to keep and what "no longer fits." We need to give ourselves credit for all of the important things that we have accomplished thus far in our lives. We also need to re-examine our priorities and change our perceptions of ourselves and others. It is time to re-evaluate our goals, our hopes, and our dreams. We must be willing to give up the fantasy of living "happily ever after" and "having it all." We must start to face the realities behind the myths. Rather than being afraid or depressed we need to ask ourselves: What now? What next?

We can begin this process by asking questions. Questions such as the following:
- How can I nurture myself?
- What do I find fulfilling?
- What are my interests?
- What am I good at? (Although, just because you are good at something doesn't mean that you must do it!)
- What is my passion? (What is it that you do that allows time to pass without your knowing it? You suddenly lookup and say, "Where has the time gone!")

Possible Areas of Reinvestment

For many women, their education was postponed or interrupted by marriage and/or childbirth. Some women sacrificed their education in order to support their families. You may want to consider <u>Investing in Education:</u>
- Start or return to college
- Learn a new trade or skill: becoming a chef, or dental hygienist, or auto mechanic

- Take a community education class
- Attend a Road Scholar program. Road Scholar is a not-for-profit organization providing "educational adventures that engage people for whom learning is the journey of a life time." Adventures range from foreign travel, to college classes, even golf and bicycling adventures. www.roadscholar.org

Have you been stuck in the same career for many years—stuck in a rut you can't seem to escape? With more time and freedom at midlife, you may choose <u>Investing in a New Career:</u>
- Start a new business
- Get retrained for a career - either one that you left behind or from which you were terminated.
- Community service work
- Non-profit work
- Part-time work

You don't necessarily have to go back to college or join the workforce at midlife. In fact, some women may choose early retirement. For many women, midlife finally gives them the time, money, and freedom for <u>Investing in a Hobby or the Arts:</u>
- Crafts: knitting, sewing, crocheting, quilting, wood working
- Performing arts: dance, acting, singing, playing an instrument
- Sports: golf, ice skating, fishing, biking, swimming, running, tennis
- Decorative Arts: painting, redecorating, ceramics, jewelry making, interior design
- Traveling to places you have always wanted to see
- Writing

Some women awaken in midlife longing for "something more." For these women, <u>Investing in the Spiritual Realm</u> may be rewarding and fulfilling:
- Traditional religion
- Non-traditional religion
- Serving others: working in a hospice or with Habitat for Humanity
- Starting an inner journey

Deciding how to reinvest

Deciding what it is we want to reinvest in may be frustrating. Sometimes it is difficult for women to even remember or recognize what gives them fulfillment or enjoyment. We have often heard women say, "It has been so long since I thought about what I want that I don't even know what I want anymore." Women spend so many years nurturing and pleasing others that they often lose touch with their own thoughts and feeling. Often women feel selfish just thinking about their own needs and desires.

To determine how we want to reinvest we need to give ourselves permission and time: permission to think about ourselves, and time for our thoughts to incubate. The following are activities that may be helpful:

- Spending time alone, often in nature
- Talking with a trusted friend
- Researching and reading
- Taking classes and workshops
- Counseling with a professional
- Meditating, yoga
- Praying
- Taking a trip or a vacation
- Engaging in playful, relaxing activities: gardening, golf, cleaning, painting, throwing a party
- Keeping a dream journal
- Brainstorming and listing your girlhood goals. What were your goals before puberty, before pleasing men and society became important?
- Brainstorming for your interests and writing them down with your non-dominant hand (left if you are right-handed, the right hand if you are left handed). Using your non-dominate hand encourages creativity, and a new way of thinking.
- Joining an online support group.

The Decision: What now?

The answer to "what now?" comes for some as an "aha!" experience. For others, it is a more gradual knowing. There can be an enormous sense of joy and release, as well as an overwhelming feeling to finally discover "who we want to be when we grow up"

Implementation

Reinvesting in our new grown up lives can be both exciting and terrifying. For some, the process is clear and direct. More often, however, knowing what we want is just the beginning. Knowing how to accomplish it becomes the new problem and involves risks.   It may even involve reinventing ourselves. No matter how we react to the idea of implementation—be it joy or fear--there can be a variety of obstacles to overcome:

Stumbling Blocks to implementation
- Lack of preparation or education
- Lack of money
- Putting others' needs before our own
- Lack of time: caring for children, grandchildren, aging parents.
- Lack of family support
- Fear of taking a risk, fear of failure
- Fear of change: it is uncomfortable and uncertain
- Lack of self esteem
- Guilt from letting go of our old, nurturing roles
- Fear of being judged as "selfish"
- Feelings of uncertainty and resignation
- Fatigue, illness

Although the stumbling blocks may seem insurmountable, overcoming them—however difficult or exhausting—is well worth the effort. Success results in a sense of satisfaction and pride, renewed energy, and new opportunities.

For some, the reinvestment process will follow a linear pattern. They will identify the goal and go for it! However, for others, it will not be so simple. It will be more like, "I thought I knew what I wanted but now I am not so sure." "Do I really want to go back to school in education, or in psychology?" " Do I really want to go back to school or continue to work on improving my golf game?" One may start to school and then have to drop out for a period of time. It will be an organic process as one shuttles back and forth through the reinvestment process

Some women may need the help of a professional such as a therapist, life coach, career counselor or even a marriage counselor to overcome stumbling blocks. Others may choose to form a small group of trusted friends and use this workbook as the focus for discussions about midlife and menopause. Journaling, keeping a diary, or just writing down your thoughts are great ways to reflect upon what is happening to you at this stage of your life. Exercise helps, too, to change our negative attitudes and overcome our fears.

Be patient with yourself. Don't beat yourself up if you set your goals too high and then have to lower them. Crises arise (deaths, illnesses, or children moving back home) that may sidetrack you temporarily. Don't get discouraged or give up. Remember, you have the rest of your life to complete this journey.

Journal Prompts/ Discussion Questions:

MIDLIFE AS A GREIF PROCESS- STAGE 4: REINVESTMENT AND REINVENTION

- ✓ Where are you in the reinvestment process?

- ✓ What have you accomplished so far in your life of which you can be proud?

- ✓ The fairytales we heard as children usually ended with, "And they lived happily ever after." What does "living happily ever after" mean to you at midlife?

- ✓ Our lives are like patchwork quilts that aren't finished yet. What new pieces will you be working on? What else would I like to accomplish with my life?   What legacy would I like to leave behind? What goals do I have yet to achieve?

- ✓ Complete several of the suggested activities listed such as brainstorming or meditating for determining your areas of possible reinvestment.

- ✓ What areas have you identified for reinvestment?

- ✓ What are your stumbling blocks?

- ✓ What are your strategies for overcoming your stumbling blocks?

- ✓ How can you use the nurturing skills you have developed to enable your own growth process?

- ✓ Continue to evaluate your progress through the reinvention process. How do you feel about the person you are becoming? Do you need to stop and reevaluate or take a "detour"? Remember this process takes time.

SECTION THREE:
Male Menopause

MALE MIDLIFE

We decided to add a short section on men and midlife because it is helpful for women to be aware of what men may be going through as well in midlife. Understanding and compassion are important in relationships during these difficult years. It has been said that midlife is the most difficult state of life for both men and women.

Andropause
Men do not experience true menopause because even after hormone changes men can remain fertile. At midlife men do however have a rebalancing of hormones that may result in symptoms. This period is referred to as andropause.

Myths of Menopause:
- *There is not such a thing as male menopause. If there are issues they are minor and will get better on their own.*

- *Male midlife problems can only be cured with hormone (testosterone)   replacement.*

Facts of Menopause:
- *Midlife for men begins around 40 and lasts until 60 (although testosterone levels continue to fall until they reach a pre-puberty level at around age 80).*

- *Men's hormones change at a much slower rate that women's therefore men typically experience fewer symptoms.*

- *Men may have some or all of the following: hot flushes, night sweats, irritability, fatigue, depression, anger, weight gain, low libido or impotence, insomnia, loss of memory, lack of concentration, broken sleep, mood swings, diminished physical strength and stamina.*

Management options
Recommendations:
A healthy life style including healthy eating, exercise, limiting alcohol and tobacco use, and reducing stress is particularly important as we age for men

and women. A quality vitamin-mineral supplement may be helpful. Increasing zinc in one's diet or with a supplement (5 -10 mg daily) is beneficial for maintaining prostate health as is the herb Saw Palmento.

Testosterone replacement has become increasingly popular of treating the symptoms of low testosterone. Hormone treatment for men, as for women, has its risks as well as benefits. If considering replacement it is important to work with a knowledgeable health professional.

Avoid:
Smoking – contributes to impotence
Alcohol- destroys nerves in the penis and contributes to prostate problems

Psychological and Emotional Concerns
Not all of mens midlife changes are due to low testosterone. Men like women are affected by psychological and emotional concerns of midlife.

Midlife Stressors and Life Changes
Men have many of the same stressful changes in midlife as women. See Holmes and Rahe Life Change index in SECTION TWO.

Midlife Blue Funk
Like women, men may also experience a Blue Funk in midlife.
Men say things like the following:
- My friends bore me.
- My wife no longer turns me on.
- I am uncertain about my ability to perform sexually.
- My children are strange and ungrateful.
- My job security feels precarious.
- I am dissatisfied in my current job.
- My financial burden is backbreaking.
- My hopes and goals seemed to have been misplaced.
- I am no longer the authority.
- Young men are taking my place

These feelings are uncomfortable; however, they are not abnormal at this stage of life. This is when men may attempt to cope with their feeling with behaviors typically associated with the men's "midlife crisis": drugs, affairs, sports cars.

Losses
Again the losses for men are similar to those of women at this stage of life.
- Death of family members
- Death of friends
- Loss of good health
- Loss of job
- Loss of youth
- Loss of virility
- Loss of power, particularly for men
- Loss of role in the household with changing roles for men and women.

Men like women must go through the grieving process of loss, denial, anger, and acceptance for their losses so that they can move on to reinvestment and reinvention. For men this means learning to value wisdom over power and to relate socially rather than sexually. It means learning mental flexibility verses mental rigidity and moving from a concern for and investment in oneself to a concern and investment in the community and future generations.

Summary
Midlife can be a difficult time for men and women. We need understanding, patience, and compassion for each other. A healthy life style is always appropriate, and talking with a counseling professional can be very helpful.

SECTION FOUR:
<u>SUMMARY</u>

SUMMARY

Midlife is a time of awakening. It is an exciting time of opportunity and taking charge and regaining control of our lives. It is a time of re-examining our experiences and piecing them together. Our marriages, our children, our careers, our families, our friends, our hobbies, our health, our finances, our losses, our achievements, our disappointments, our joys, our successes, our failures, our gifts, our weaknesses, our hopes, our dreams all are different pieces of our own unique patchwork quilt.

Midlife is a time for grieving our losses, re-examining our lives, letting go of what no longer works, and reinvesting that energy to build on our strengths and find meaning in the rest of our lives. We need to give ourselves permission to enjoy this stage of our lives.

It is important to get the facts, to know the realities of menopause versus the myths. It is also important to know ourselves: our strengths and vulnerabilities. Many of midlife's health changes can be managed with a good attitude and simple lifestyle changes. Menopause is just one more patch to be worked into the rest of our quilt. It has rough edges that are smoothed over with time and patience. We should live our lives without guilt and without obsessing over all of the latest and sometimes incorrect and often conflicting health advice. We do not want to become one more of the "worried well."

Use this workbook and a journal to keep in touch with the new woman you are in the process of becoming. Use the Reading List and Resources to continue learning and growing. Participate in, or start your own discussion group, like a quilting circle, for sharing your experiences, empowering, encouraging, and educating one another. Knowledge is powerful, and social support is essential to our well-being.

SECTION FIVE:
<u>Appendix</u>

GLOSSARY

Depression:

> **Every day blues**: Spirits are low, reduced drive, general feeling of pessimism

> **Grief Depression**: Reaction to a traumatic event such as the loss of a loved one. The world seems impoverished. Guilt, as well as, sleep disturbances and tears are experienced. Six weeks to six months for resolution.

> **Clinical Depression**: Lack of drive, loss of pleasure, fatigue, helplessness, suicidal thoughts and acts. Needing the care of a mental health professional.

ERT: Estrogen Replacement Therapy

Estrogen: General term for the female sex hormones

> **E1 or Estrone**: One form of estrogen. One of the main components of birth control pills and HRT (Hormone Replacement Therapy). Converted in the liver to Estriol.
> **E2 or Estradiol**: Most potent form of estrogen. One of the main components of birth control pills and HRT, along with Estrone. Most stimulating to the breast. The more potent the estrogen, the more possibility it has of causing side effects, endometrial cancer and possibly breast cancer.
> **E3 or Estriol**: The form of estrogen most active in the vagina, cervix, and vulva. Estriol is the main estrogen in the body when women are pregnant. The weakest form of estrogen; it is considered to be anti-carcinogenic (anti-cancer producing).

Formication: A sensation associated with menopause of having insects crawling all over one's skin.

Follicle-Stimulating Hormone (FSH): The hormone that initiates the growth of follicles (eggs) within the ovaries.

HRT: Hormone Replacement Therapy using both estrogen and progestin.

Kegel Exercise: Kegel exercise is for strengthening the pelvic-floor muscles that support the urethra, bladder, uterus, and rectum. Doing them often and correctly can improve muscle strength, thereby improving urine control and increasing sexual response. To isolate these muscles trying stopping and starting the flow of urine. Once you have located them squeeze for 4 counts and then release for 4 counts. Try to do this exercise for 5 minutes twice a day. At first, you may not be able to do it for 5 minutes at one time, but like any exercise, it will get easier with time.

Luteinizing Hormone (LH): The hormone that stimulates estrogen secretion and stimulates the ovary to secrete progesterone following ovulation.

Menopause: The single point in time of the last menstrual period

Surgical Menopause: Menopause beginning immediately following the surgical removal of both ovaries. Women who have only one ovary removed can expect to go through a normal menopause except possibly at a younger age.

Medical Menopause: Menopause as a result of the use of a drug (often Tamoxifen) prescribed to stop estrogen production for women with a medical condition such as breast cancer.

Osteoporosis: A reduction in the density of the skeleton: a loss of bone mass and increased fragility often resulting in factures.

Perimenopause: The stage in the aging process of women marking the transition form the reproductive state of life to the non-reproductive state. Perimenopause is a gradual process. The decline in estrogen usually takes four to five years. It can begin as early as age 35 or be delayed as late as 50.

Phytohormones: Hormones found in plants that help the human body produce its own natural estrogen and progesterone. They are 1/400 as potent as human estrogen. They are often effective in relieving menopausal symptoms. It is thought that phytohormones take up the estrogen receptor sites in the body, thereby causing the more potent estrogens to be excreted.   Below is a list of natural sources of phytohormones:

Alfalfa	Cherries	Licorice	Rice
Almonds	Coffee	Oats	Rye
Anise	Corn	Parsley	Sage
Apples	Fennell	Peas	Sesame
Barley	French Beans	Peanuts	Soy beans-tofu
Black Cohash	Garlic	Pomegranates	Wheat
Carrots	Ginseng	Potatoes	
Cashew nuts	Green Beans	Red Beans	

Postmenopause: The phase of a women's life beginning one year after her last menstrual period.

Progesterone: A hormone produced by the ovary and released following ovulation necessary for preparing the uterus and breast for pregnancy and for the production and regulation of certain other steroid hormones including estrogen and testosterone.

Progestins: Term for synthetic hormone substances like Provera that produce effects similar to those of natural progesterone.

READING LIST

Balch, Phyllis A. . *Prescription for Nutritional Healing.* 5rd Ed. New York: Penguin Group, 2010.

A nutritional approach to menopause and other conditions with specific, easy-to-use recommendations.

Barnes, Broda O., and Lawrence Galton. *Hypothyroidism: The Unsuspected Illness.* New York: Harper & Row, 1990.

Still the definitive work on hypothyroidism and its far-reaching effects, including a simple, do it yourself test for thyroid function.

Barbach, Lonnie. *The Pause.* New York: Plume, 2000.

A highly recommended, useful reference covering all aspects of menopause.

Beck, Martha. *Finding Your Own North Star.* New York: 3 Rivers Press, 2001.

A step-by-step program that will lead your to your own best life.

Brown, Brene. *"The Midlife Unraveling".* May 24, 2018. www.*brenebrown.com*

Calhoun, Ana. *"The New Midlife Crisis: Why and How it is Hitting Gen X Women."* www.*Oprah.com*

Cohen, Gene D. *The Mature Mind: The Positive Power of the Aging Brain.* New York: Basic, 2005.

An encouraging book about the how the human brain grows and flourishes rather than simply declining in the second half of life.

Crook, W. G. *The Yeast Connection and Women*. Jackson: Professional, 1995.

Diamond, Jed. *Surviving Male menopause. A Guide for Women and Men.* Naperville: Sourcebooks, Inc., 2001.

Gaby, Alan R. *Preventing and Reversing Osteoporosis*. Roseville: Roma, 1995.

Information on osteoporosis research. Gaby argues that not only is osteoporosis preventable without medication, but it can also be reversed.

Gittleman, Ann Louise. *Hot times: How to Eat Well, Live Healthy, and Feel Sexy During the Change.* New York: Avery, 2005.

Gittleman shows how to control menopause symptoms safely and naturally with her detoxify nutritional program.

Hahn, Linaya. *PMS and Menopause: Solving the Puzzle: Sixteen Causes of Premenstrual Syndrome and What to Do About It* , Soquel, CA, Empowered Whole Being Press. 2015.

An excellent discussion of factors that affect our hormones and brain chemistry. Informative and helpful, as well as easy to read. Useful in menopause because often PMS symptoms become worse. Some have described menopause as chronic PMS. Also includes a useful discussion on yeast problems and thyroid problems.

Lee, John. *What Your Doctor May Not Tell You About Menopause.* New York: Time Warner, 1996.

This is the Dr. Lee's work supporting and promoting the use of natural progesterone.

Martin, Raquel with Judi Gerstung. ***The Estrogen Alternative: Natural Hormone Therapy with Botanical Progestrone***. 3rd edition. Rochester: Healing Arts Press. 2000.

Nelson, Miriam. ***Strong Women Stay Young.*** New York: Bantam, 2005.
  A useful reference on exercise for women.

Northrup, Christiane. ***The Wisdom of Menopause.*** New York: Bantam, 2012.

Norsigian, Judy and Vivian Pinn. ***Our Bodies, Ourselves: Menopause.*** New York: Touchstone, 2006.

  This book is written in cooperation with the Boston Women's Health Book Collective. A contemporary look at women and aging. It includes an extensive resource guide for information, services, and organizations.

Seaman, Barbara, and Laura Eldridge. ***The no-nonsense guide to menopause.*** Simon and Schuster. 2008.

  A comprehensive resource with simple, unbaiased advice on managing this menopause including a thorough discusion on the HRT decision.

Sanson, Gillian. ***The Myth of Osteoporosis.*** Ann Arbor, MI: MCD Century Publications, 2003.
  Provides clear insight into the myths of osteoporosis and invaluable knowledge for creating as well as maintaining bone health. It gives

women good reasons for challenging the common way that osteoporosis is handled in the United States.

Sheehy, Gail. *Sex and the Seasoned Woman: Pursuing the Pasionate Life.* New York: Random House, 2006.

Sheehey always has an interesting perspective or the stages of life.

Somers, Suzanne. *Ageless: The Naked Truth About Bioidentical Hormones.* New York: Crown, 2006

A detailed discussion of the treatment of menopause with the use of bioidentical hormones. Good glossary and resource section.

Warga, Claire. *Menopause and the Mind.* NV: Free Press, 2000.

An interesting read for those who think they may be losing their minds.

Warshowsky, Allan, and Elena Oumano. *Healing Fibroids: A doctor's Guide to a Natural Cure.* New York: Fireside, 2002.

Weed, Susan S. New *Menopausal Years: The Wise Woman Way: Alternative Approaches for Women 30—90.* Woodstock: Ash Tree, 2002.

A step-by-step guide for managing the symptoms of menopause using herbs, vitamins, meditation, and other non-medical resources.

Wentz, Izabella. *Hashimoto's Thyroiditis: Lifestyle Intervention for Finding and Testing the Root Cause.* 1st edition. San Francisco: Harper One, 2017.

An alternative explanation and good reference for those with difficult to treat thyroid problems.

RESOURCES

There are numerous resources available online. When searching, however, be sure to double-check your sources reliability. Be aware of who is sponsoring the page; i.e. is it a pharmaceutical or manufacturer promoting their own philosophy and products.

Here are a few reccomended resources.

Donna S. Kohlhepp RN, Ph.D.
201 Beaver Dr.
DuBois, PA 15801
814-375-2750
Follow on Facebook: @Dr.DonnaK
Health consulting by appointment (phone or office visit). Supplements and products available on site or by mail.

HERS Foundation
422 Bryn Mawr Ave.
Bala Cynwyd, PA 19004
610-667-7757
www.hersfoundation.com
A foundation devoted to preventing unnecessary hysterectomies by giving women information to make information decisions. Counseling is also available for women experiencing problems as a result of a hysterectomy.

Jaynes robes
www.jaynesrobe.com Beautiful robes for those undergoing breast cancer treatment.

National Women's Health Network
514 10th Street NW   Suite 400
Washington, DC 20004
202-347-1140
www.nwhn.org
A network membership organization that promotes women's health. Information packets are available on various topics such as the following: hormone therapy, fibroids, cancer. A good source of unbiased information.

Thyroid information
wwwThyroid-info.com
>*Useful information and resources for dealing with thyroid disorders, as well as, a list of Top Docs reommended by readers.*

Izabella Wentz
www.thryoidpharmacist.com
Articles, resources and supplements for dealing with Hashimoto's.

Women's International Pharmacy
5708 Monona Drive
Madison, WI 53716-3152
1-800-279-5708
www.womensinternational.com
A good beginning source of information on natural hormone replacement. Products are available by prescription. Hotline consultations are also available.

About the authors

Donna Sell Kohlhepp is a women's health consultant specializing in menopause and thyroid disorders. She earned her doctorate in Public Health at the University of Oklahoma where she also earned her Masters of Science in Community Health Nursing. Donna earned her Bachelors of Science in Nursing at The Ohio State University. As a health care consultant and educator for over 30 years Dr. Kohlhepp has not only written and done research but also directed numerous seminars and workshops from a holistic prespective. Donna is married to Daniel B. Kohlhepp, PhD. They have three daughters: Kaydee Gunter, Joanne Bish, and Kimberly Kohlhepp. Dan and Donna live in Arlington, Virginia and DuBois, Pennsylvania.

Jayne M. Magee is a retired professor of English at Lakeland Community College in Kirtland, Ohio. Jayne earned her doctorate in Rhetoric and Linguistics at Indiana University of Pennsylvania. She earned her BA in English at the University of Missouri and her MA in English at Clarion University of Pennsylvania. Jayne teaches weaving and knitting. Jayne is married to Gary Magee,DC, and they have four children: Meghan, Mandy, Gabe, and Galen. Jayne and Gary live in DuBois, Pennsylvania. Jayne teaches weaving and knitting at Amy's Yarn Boutique, does feelance editing, and writes in her spare time.